# HOW TO CURE ECZEMA IN KIDS

## *MIRACLE REMEDIES THAT REALLY WORK*

By

*ANNE WORTHINGTON*

Copyright © 2018

# INTRODUCTION

Eczema is a debilitating skin condition that can dramatically affect the sufferer's quality of life. But I'm going to share with you the simple remedies that cured severe eczema for both my daughters.

But I'll be clear on this: when I say "cure", I mean my all visible signs of it were completely gone. Not even a minor rash. But it does not mean my daughters genes have been modified, and eczema appears to be a permanent condition. So if my daughters were to stop the remedies we're using, their eczema would return. For example, giving them too much chocolate always results in a rash. So they only get chocolate at Easter, and not too much of it.

**The answer is not steroid creams or drugs, which do provide temporary relief but are not a permanent solution.**

**If you follow the simple instructions in this book, you'll see an enormous improvement in your condition.**

# ABOUT THIS BOOK

My two daughters had severe eczema since they were babies. The doctors mostly offered temporary solutions such as creams and drugs, which came with significant warnings and side-effects.

Believe me they're not the answer. They're a temporary remedy.

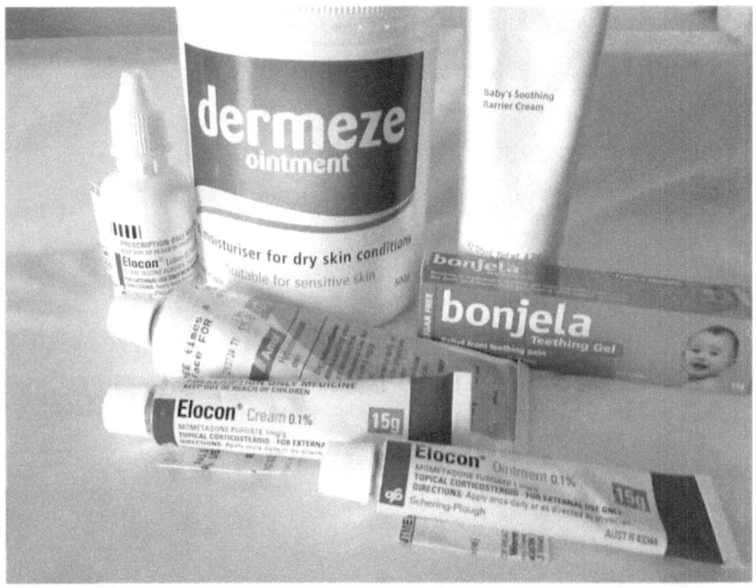

While I do believe in modern medicine, I also believe doctors are often too quick to prescribe drugs. In particularly with eczema, the solutions are much simpler than you'd think.

When my daughters were referred to skin specialists, they advised a range of treatments which did work to a degree, but were not a complete solution. And the ongoing appointments with specialists were costing a fortune.

The best long-term solution came from lots of research, advice from doctors and skin specialists, and trial and error. Yes unfortunately there's some trial and error involved too, because everyone's body is slightly different. Still it all comes back to the same principles I explain.

Although lots of the advice I give in this book came from qualified specialists, I suggest not relying on this book alone. It is probably everything you need because specialists will likely give you the same advice, but it is wiser to see a doctor just in case.

I wrote this book to explain everything that works.

But understand I'm not a writer. And I don't believe in long books with useless information so I'll keep everything short and concise.

# Verifying Advice Accuracy

Especially when it comes to medical advice, never take someone's word alone. So in this book I'll provide both the advice, and the references at the end.

The reality is I've used a large variety of sources to find solutions that worked for my daughters, but at least the sources I provide show you the solutions work for others, rather than just my daughters.

The resources will also give you valuable advice, but it's also included in this book anyway.

# TREATMENTS FROM THE DOCTORS & SPECIALISTS

Again I'm not a doctor. I'm just a mother who did their own research to find permanent solutions for her daughters. The advice I give does include the same advice from specialists, but you should not rely on this alone. I suggest seeing a specialist because there might be factors not covered in this book.

Now let's start with how it began for my daughters, and the medical advice we received.

During the colder months, both my daughters became covered in rashes – in particularly in the folds of skin such as behind the knees. It would seem to spread like an infection, so at first we didn't know what it was. Of course I had my suspicions, but a diagnosis from the doctor confirmed it.

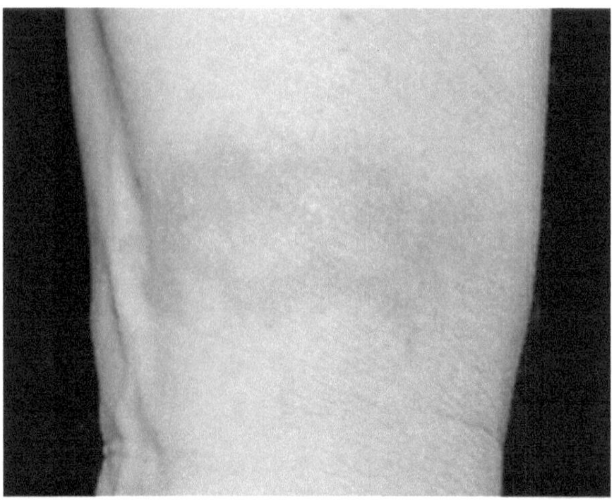

Besides some general advice, steroid creams were prescribed. We had a try a few different types before we found some that worked.

Some of the creams didn't work at all, and some made an amazing difference even within a 24hr period. If you use a cream and the improvements are not noticeable within a few days, try another cream. But remember the creams are still just a temporary solution for when rashes really flare up.

If you are persistent with seeing doctors and specialists, it will cost a lot of money but you will usually get all the solutions you need. Hopefully this book will help you avoid that.

Be aware though, don't rely on just the opinion and advice of one practitioner. This is because many are quite lazy, and will only give you general advice, with a heavy reliance on creams.

I find the majority of doctors tend to treat the symptoms, rather than address the cause of conditions. Perhaps this is because the medical industry is largely about pharmaceutical companies and selling drugs. But I want to appear pessimistic or negative, but I believe doctors are way too quick to prescribe drugs.

On the other hand, many holistic practitioners tend to rely too heavily on herbs and natural therapies. I believe the answer varies between different people, so what works for one person won't necessarily work for another.

Probably the most common example of doctors treating the symptoms instead of addressing the cause is everyday painkillers. The most common painkiller simply blocks the message of pain reaching your brain, but does nothing to address the cause. Plus it has a nasty side affect of harming your liver.

# IRRITANTS AND ALLERGENS

Now let's look at the causes of eczema, and how to be rid of it once and for all.

But keep in mind the solution is not a magic pill you swallow. What works for one person will not necessarily work for another. So you will need to be patient, and trial and error is involved.

It also helps to keep a logbook especially if the condition is particularly bad. This is because you need to know what may be causing the problems.

# SOAPS

It doesn't take much to irritate sensitive skin. Some soap can severely dehydrate skin. Most of the time you can find suitable soap at your local grocery store. Don't rely too much on so packaging, because not everything that goes into soap is listed on the packages.

As a general rule, use unscented soaps with no artificial additives. I have had the most success with goat milk soap, which is usually something you need to order through the Internet.

Below is a list of specific brands you can try, which should be available in your local grocery store.

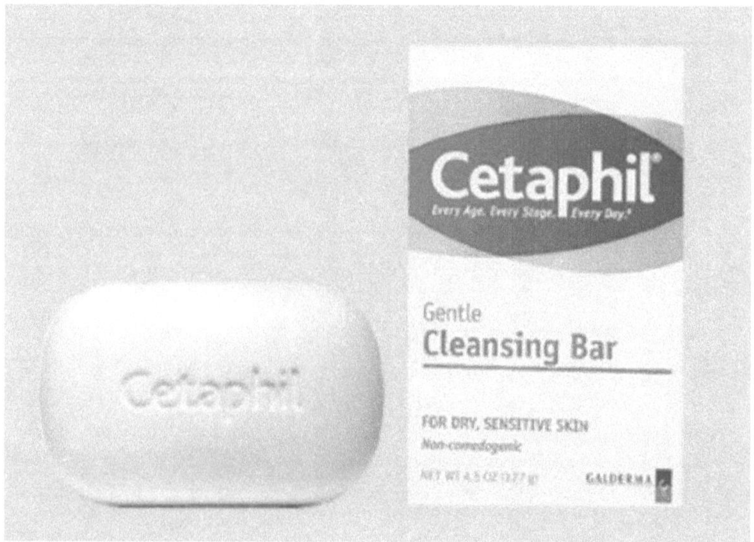

**Aveeno Body Wash.**

This is more for adults, as it's not something you put in the bath. One of the ingredients is oatmeal, which is particularly good at helping to repair the skin barrier. Part of the reason harsh soaps cause eczema to worsen is because it degrades the skin barrier, making the rash more likely to break out.

Many products with oatmeal also include harsh chemicals that counteract the benefits. Carefully check additives.

**Dove Unscented For Sensitive Skin.**

Dove is a very widely available brand of soap. You can buy it just about anywhere in the world.

What makes it particularly good is that some variants are pH neutral, meaning it is neither acidic or alkaline. You can buy very cheap pH test strips from eBay. Simply lay a test strip on a wet bar of soap, and follow the test strip procedures to determine the pH.

**Goat Milk Soap.**

Goat milk soap is probably easiest for children. It is widely available on the Internet in places such as eBay, but you may need to try a few different suppliers. Again I recommend using pH test strips and give preference to suppliers who soap is either pH neutral, or with a higher pH, meaning the soap is slightly alkaline. Slightly alkaline is better because your body is slightly alkaline.

It's best to purchase the powdered form of goat soap, so you can add a few scoops to the water in a bath.

**Cetaphil Skin Cleanser.**

This is another product more intended for adults. It is generally used without water, such as a bath or shower. Generally you use it if you need to clean places like your face.

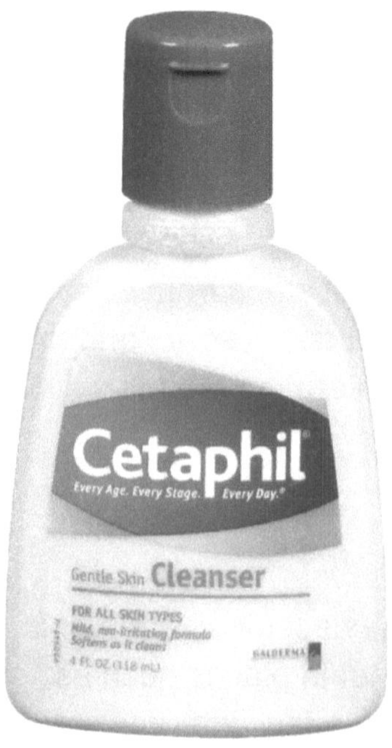

# Detergents

The detergent you use to wash clothes will contact your skin all day. You can easily find detergents suitable for sensitive skins, but they still almost always have fragrances that alone can cause irritation. So again you may need to try a few different brands.

On the note of washing clothes, you may have low-irritant clothing for a child with eczema, but still wash their clothes with other clothes. And the dyes from other clothes may be causing a problem. So be attentive to clothes you are washing together.

At the very least, wash any new clothes before wearing them.

# BUBBLE BATHS.

Bubble baths can be a nightmare for children with eczema. They are usually made from cheap ingredients which are particularly harsh on the skin. Cheaper and harsher chemicals tend to strip protective coating from skin, and make it more prone to rash breakout.

But at the same time you don't want to deny your children the fun of a bubble bath. It's not something you do every bath, at least it wasn't when I was a child. So below I have listed some brands which are much less harsh than what you normally buy from shops.

**Trukid Bubble Podz.**

This is a bubble bath specifically with eczema in mind. It contains oatmeal, Aloe Vera, and vitamin E. It is unscented, but still gives plenty of bubbles for kids to play in.

I have tried a variety of different brands, which have much the same ingredients. But it really pays to have simple pH test strips you can get from eBay. Again you want to avoid anything that is too acidic.

**Child's Farm Bubble Bath For Sensitive Skin.**

This is one brand of bubble bath where mothers of sufferers are raving about it. I haven't tried it personally because I haven't needed to, but if your child loves bubble baths, it's something to try.


**General Advice About Bubble Wash.**

Adding some eczema-friendly body wash will add bubbles to the water, but it's an expensive way to go about it.

If you can't find a suitable bubble bath mixture, generally you can use whatever you find at the store. But after the bath, rinse the child in the shower to ensure all suds are off them. Then use appropriate moisturizer on the skin later. It's not something you can do all the time, because strong chemicals will affect the skin despite any attempts to repair it later on with moisturizers.

Most of the suitable bubble wash products don't have any coloring. This makes it a little more boring for your child, and you wouldn't want to rob them of colored bath. You can add a very small amount of colored food dye, but be very careful with it because it can stain everything from your fingers to clothes. And if you leave the water sitting in the bath too long, you can actually stain the acrylic of your bath which is nearly impossible to get out.

This is the same case with other colored bubble baths, whether they are suitable for eczema sufferers or not. In fact I left colored water in the bath for about an hour, and now the bath is permanently stained. It might not show one a colored bath tub, but it certainly does on white.

**Avoiding Hot Baths.**

One guaranteed way to flare up eczema is to have a hot bath or shower. Having your skin to hot will have the same effect. Bath or shower water should be not much warmer than lukewarm.

For some people, this may be the only solution you need. In fact I had a friend with severe eczema all through his childhood, even into high school. His rashes were particularly bad especially behind the knees. And one day I noticed it was gine. I asked him how he cured it, and he said all he needed to do was to have cooler showers. He said his findings were eczema is actually a blood condition rather than a skin condition.

My experience with my daughters is even irritating the skin over short periods of time with higher temperatures is enough to cause flare-ups. So you can't simply give your child a hot bath, and end it by adding cool water. The damage will have already been done. If lukewarm water makes no difference, try having a slightly cooler bath or shower.

# SHAMPOOS.

Shampoo is an irritant that is easily overlooked. Even just hair conditioner could be part of the problem, but you don't normally think about it. Especially in a child's bath, anything you put on their hair will end up in the water and ultimately on and in their skin.

There are a variety of shampoos that are friendly to eczema sufferers, but they are less common than various soaps. Presumably this is because most people don't link a hair product to a skin condition.

Again test the pH of the shampoo to ensure it is either neutral or slightly alkaline. Generally if a shampoo is scented, it won't be friendly to eczema sufferers.

The more you do research on shampoos, the more you come to understand there's a lot that goes into them that you don't suspect.

Avoid shampoos with salicylic acid and ketoconazole. But there are far too many other additives to mention. As always, give preference to shampoos which are specifically designed for eczema sufferers. You also need to consider such shampoos may be fine for adults, but not good for kids when they get it in their eyes. You don't always know how painful it may be for a child with each new brand. Just keep a clean face wash towel nearby so you can dry your child's eyes if needed.

Three brands I recommend are Neutragena, Exederm and Dermaveen. At least these are two I have had good results with. But again I must remind you that what works for one person does not necessarily work for another. So try a variety of different brands, and carefully note the results. In most cases you only need to use it a few times to know if there's any difference. It's also important to keep a logbook so you know what has been changed. If you change several different things at once, it makes it very difficult to determine what's working and what's not working. Or even what has made the problem worse.

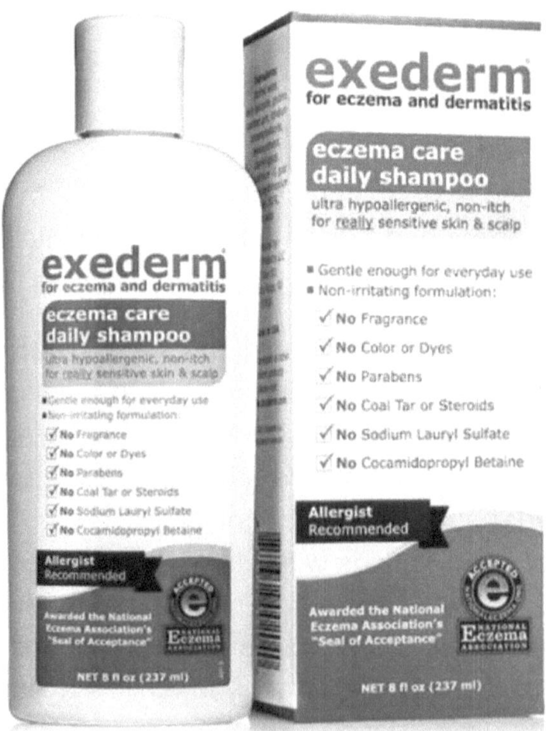

# Clothing.

The wrong clothing can be a persistent disaster for eczema. When it's cold, it's easy to tell your kids to wrap up warm. But if you wear too much you can get sweaty. And when sweat remains on your skin, it is bound to make eczema worse. Of course it's okay to stay warm, but avoid getting too warm. You just want to be at a point where you are not cold, but you are comfortable.

In particularly keep in mind that the majority of your body heat is lost through your neck and head. So covering up your torso and arms in order to stay warm may not be best. Consider wearing a beanie instead. This way your arms and legs can breathe better, and be less prone to sweating.

You need clothing to be breathable so it can keep you warm, but allow any sweat to dry.

**Suitable Materials.**

Overall the best material is cotton, because it breathes. Carefully check the labels on clothing before purchasing.

Any synthetic material is a bad idea. But also wool, which is completely natural, tends to irritate the skin and worsen eczema.

**Summer Clothing.**

You'll probably notice that eczema clears up more in the summer. This is because the skin is allowed to breathe, and there is nothing touching the skin if you are wearing shorts.

The only downside to the summer is suncream is a huge irritant. Even the supposedly eczema friendly suncreams can be serious irritants. There is no real way around this. In the summer, you don't want to wear clothing in the summer heat. And you don't want to need suncream. My suggestion is you suncream, but only brands that are designed for eczema sufferers. And when you are out of the sun, don't leave the cream on you. Use one of the gentle soaps to clean it off your skin. Don't use any harsh chemicals of soaps because it will damage the surface of your skin, making you more prone to breakouts.

**Bedding and sheets.**

Only use 100% pure cotton sheets and doona covers. Avoid anything else.

**Avoid Tight Clothes.**

Even with cotton material, clothing touching skin tends to irritate it. Even if it's 100% pure cotton.

Avoid clothing with harsh feeling seems, and carefully remove any tags. Anything that feels scratchy on the clothes will irritate your skin more.

**Use Suitable PJs.**

We'll spend a lot of time in bed, so carefully consider the pyjamas you wear. Just like your daytime close, give preference to loosefitting and cotton pyjamas. If the weather permits, use short pyjamas. The fewer clothes you wear, the better.

There are a variety of online stores that specialize in clothing for eczema sufferers. Try eczemacompany.com/eczema-clothing/ which has everything you need and even caters for children. Screenshot is below:

# Gentle Clothing

We carry **soft, soothing eczema clothing** for babies, children, teenagers and adults.

- Protective mittens to **prevent scratching.**
- Wet wrapping garments to **calm the skin.**
- Pajamas in cooling fabrics and with flat seams.

Our clothing works best when worn over top our gentle eczema cream and bath products.

**Shop our Eczema Clothing below.**

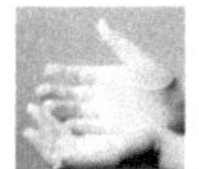

Mittens & Gloves

Remedywear
Hand Dermatitis
Gloves

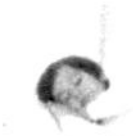

Sleepwear/Pajamas

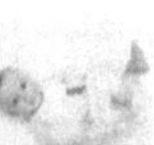

Sleeping Sacks

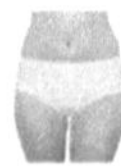

Underwear

Socks

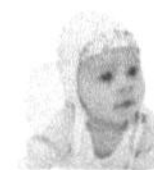

Hats

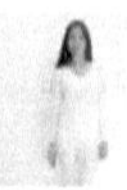

Dry Wraps

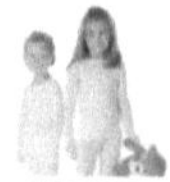

Wet Wraps

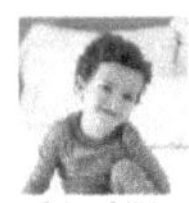

Babies & Kids

# GRASS.

You might not think something organic and natural like grass could be a problem. But even I flareup with rashes if I roll around in the grass. One particular time I merely rubbed my eye, and my whole eyelid became massively swollen. It was an allergic reaction in this case, which since hasn't been repeated. Although even just laying on grass now tends to give me rashes up and down my arms.

Both my daughters have similar reactions after playing in the grass. The rashes tend to be slightly different though, with more of our redness in the skin over a large area.

# MOISTURIZER.

You should be using a suitable moisturizer after every bath or shower. This may be a short mention, but it's very important. Keep your skin hydrated.

The good news is there are many different moisturizers designed for eczema sufferers. So you will have no trouble finding it in the local chemist or supermarket.

QV is a product we use, which was recommended by our skin specialist. The only downside is don't let your kids jump on your couch after lathering them, because there something in the cream that tends to stain in the couch.

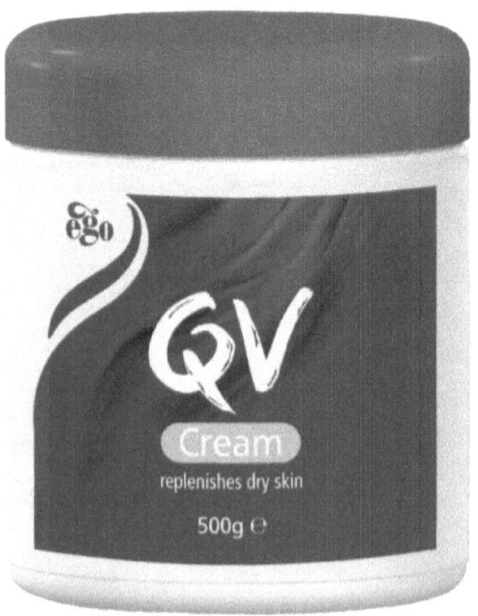

# Immune Deficiency.

None of the doctors we saw even mentioned the immune system. So we never gave much thought to it. Only with further research did we come to understand the condition become significantly worse when your immune system is weakened.

This is particularly in the colder months where you have less sunlight and may be vitamin D deficient.

There are many things you can do to boost your immune system, with the simplest below:

**Probiotics.**

These are basically good bacteria for your digestive system. If you have an unhealthy digestive system, your entire body will suffer.

You can purchase them even from your local supermarket, but you will find higher quality products from your local chemist. Specifically ask for broad-spectrum versions, with the aim of helping the digestive system and specifically the immune system.

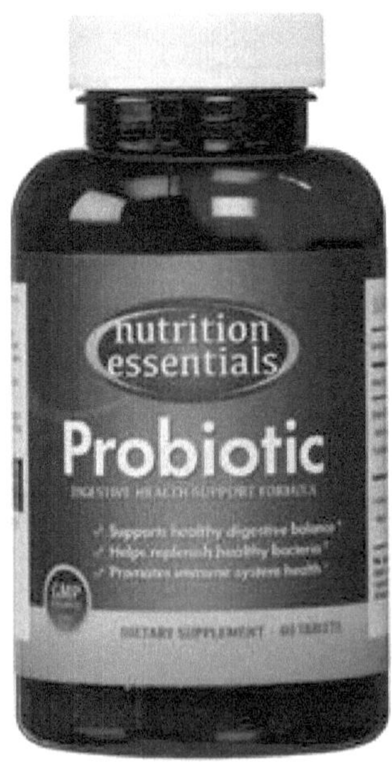

## Regular Exercise.

You should do at least 30-60 minutes of exercise per day, where your heart rate is elevated. If you don't break a sweat at all, you're probably not doing enough exercise. Ideally you should be doing even more exercise You'll also feel much better after excerise.

This is not so much a factor with children, but more so with adults. If you have a problem doing enough exercise, or perhaps find it boring, find a way to make it interesting. Ideally exercise should be an activity like riding a bike, and not feel like exercise.

**Maintain a Healthy Weight.**

Being either under or overweight will affect your immune system and overall health. There is no major secret to maintaining healthy weight. It's just a matter of eating the right foods, not too much food, and doing regular exercise.

**Get Proper Sleep.**

Nobody can function without proper sleep. Otherwise you can't think straight, and your body won't function correctly. We can all get by with limited sleep, but just "getting by" is not healthy. You should have seven or more hours of proper sleep. And by proper sleep, I mean uninterrupted and comfortable sleep.

If you aren't getting proper sleep, find and fix the problem. It could be as simple as changing pillows. You may also want to try subtle herbs such as valerian root. In particularly bad cases, try a sleep therapist.

**Immune Boosting Herbs.**

A few different herbs mixed in with cooking generally aren't even noticed, but can make a significant difference to your immune system and health.

They aren't a magic solution, and are just part of the overall picture. A list of the herbs I use most is below:

- Cayenne Pepper
- Cinnamon
- Clove
- Garlic
- Ginger
- Tumeric
- Rosemary

# VITAMIN SUPPLEMENTS.

Generally foods that contain nutrients and vitamin C are better than supplements. But you can use the following supplements:

## Vitamin D

In the cooler months I suggest regularly taking vitamin D supplements. All you usually need is the maintenance dose on a daily basis. You don't need it during the summer unless you never get outside.

## Zinc

The best form is zinc is zinc gluconate. You can get it from most chemists. Sometimes you can have it ordered in. You can also find it online.

## Omega-3

Omega 3 is best in fish, but you can also purchase supplements.

# PURE EPSOM SALT.

Epson salts are very easy to use for children because they can be placed in baths. It may be addressing the symptoms rather than the cause, but they significantly reduce the persistent itch all over your body.

It is essentially magnesium and sulphate combined, and it looks like ordinary salt. It easily dissolves in water.

Usually Epsom salt is available in your local grocery store, but often they include a variety of other chemicals for a nice scent. Avoid any Epsom salt with such additives, use only pure Epsom salt. The exception is when the additive are specifically to help eczema, such as the product below:

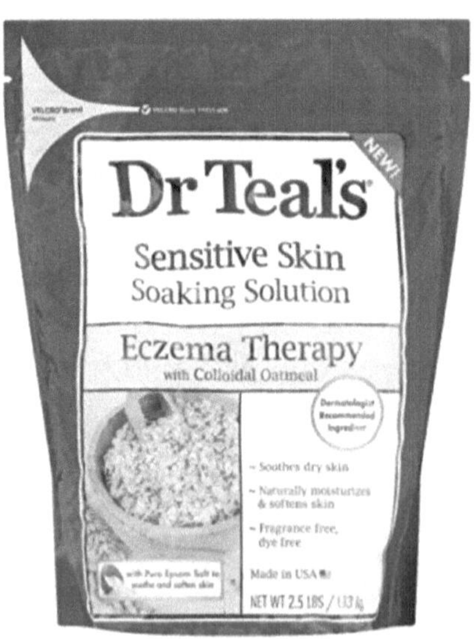

This product is made in the USA so it is more expensive if you live elsewhere. But you can easily copy the product's ingredients by adding oatmeal to pure Epsom salt.

## POLLENS.

Pollens are seasonal and can either have no noticeable effect on a sufferer, or can make a major difference. While they can be easily avoided if you are indoors, it's not realistic to live in a cave.

But you can be aware of wind direction on particular days, or if wind is strong. On days with stronger wind, limit your exposure to the outdoors.

You can use antihistamines if you are adversely affected by pollens, but usually they come with the side effect of drowsiness.

Depending on where you live, there may be websites that can even warn you about high risk days for pollen. On such days, it may be wiser to stay indoors. These websites are designed more for severe asthma sufferers.

# HOUSEHOLD PETS.

Our doctors said eczema is not an allergy, and they didn't even mention pets as a possible irritant. Initially we had two cats in our house. They were indoor cats enjoying the good life. And one of my daughters quite frequently had nasal congestion. We didn't initially consider the possibilities of the cats being irritant.

Eventually information we found online indicated it could be one of the causes, or at least an irritant. Needless to say, now the cats now live outdoors, except at night time when we lock them in the laundry. And since then, my daughter's nasal congestion simply doesn't happen anymore. It is difficult to say if the cats had any effect on her eczema, but certainly it had an effect on one of my daughters nasal congestion.

# Foods To Eat

Eating certain foods can trigger an immune system response, which leads to inflammation and ultimately eczema. The diet to help with eczema is similar to an anti-inflammatory diet. Foods that help are listed below:

**Fish.**

Fish are a natural source of omega-3, and help to reduce information. Particularly high sources include salmon, tuna, mackerel, sardines and herring.

**Probiotics.**

You can purchase these directly from your local supermarket or chemist. They essentially balance and promote intestinal health. Some yoghurts specifically contain probiotics, which may make it easier to medicate your child.

**Some fruits and vegetables.**

I say some fruits and vegetables, because some will help, and some result in a flareup every time. Fruits and vegetables to include are apples, broccoli, cherries, spinach and kale.

# FOODS TO AVOID.

Eating the wrong foods is a sure way to worsen eczema. You don't always know exactly which foods are triggering response, so it does take trial and error. But the foods listed below all have a very pronounced and definite effect, and should be avoided.

**Citrus fruits.**

If either of my daughters have oranges, within hours they are covered in rashes.

**Dairy.**

Usually a little bit of dairy is okay, but be careful to limit intake. This includes cheese.

**Eggs.**

Eggs are otherwise very healthy and beneficial. You can have them, but again limit intake.

**Gluten or wheat.**

One of my daughters is noticeably affected after having too much bread, and the other is not affected at all. I personally think that additives in bread and related products itself may be irritant.

**Soy milk or soy products.**

My daughter which is also affected by gluten and wheat tends to develop breathing difficulties after soy products, and develops new rashes. It doesn't seem to affect my other daughter.

**Tomatoes.**

Tomatoes have much the same effect as oranges with my daughters, although not as severe. Your child may not eat tomatoes directly, but they are very common. Just about every pizza pace is laced with tomato paste.

The following list of foods also have an adverse effect, although generally only to people with eczema mostly on hands and feet. This appears to be related with a heightened sensitivity to nickel. Foods that are high in nickel include:

- Beans
- black tea
- canned meats

- chocolate
- lentils
- nuts
- peas
- seeds
- shellfish
- soybeans

In many cases, foods or specific brands of food may contain additives that worsen your condition. You can carefully check additives on packages, but that alone doesn't reveal everything in them. So if you're really having trouble finding what works, try different brands.

# SUMMARY AND CONCLUSION.

Factors that flare-up eczema for one individual may have no effect on another. Everyone's bodies are slightly different, so it is important to maintain logs of products that are used, and foods that are eaten. This is the best way to determine what causes flare-ups.

For my daughters, it was a combination of typical causes. For example, we quickly learned that after Easter chocolate, flare-ups were inevitable. We would rather not completely deny our daughters the pleasure of chocolate. So simply when they had any chocolate at all, we would give them an Epsom salt bath, and a lather them with moisturizer. In this case, it was the patch job rather than a proper solution. A proper solution would be to have them avoid chocolate completely. They did have severe eczema when everything wrong was being done. But ultimately to cure it involved a variety of simple changes, and some trial and error.

Over the course of the years, we tried countless different solutions and changes that some people swore by. But again everyone is different.

At times it may feel like an uphill battle, especially as there are so many irritants you need to consider. But as we found, you may find the solution is relatively simple. Even if you don't completely eliminate rashes, with moderate care you can still expect a significant difference. How vigilant you need to be more depends on how severe the eczema is, and what is causing it.

Generally if something contacting the skin is causing an issue, skin will become red and inflamed very quickly (within an hour or so).

If something is consumed which is causing the problem, the effect many manifest in anywhere from 1-12 hours.

Because of the relatively short time-frames, it is not too difficult to track what triggers the eczema. Then it's more a matter of finding practical solutions that work for both sufferers, and the whole family.

# REFERENCES

This section lists some of the resources I've used. The list is nowhere near exhaustive though, and represents only a fraction of my sources.

alenta, R., Mittermann, I., Werfel, T., Garn, H. and Renz, H., 2009. Linking allergy to autoimmune disease. Trends in immunology, 30(3), pp.109-116.

Kimata, H., 2001. Fatty liver in atopic dermatitis. Allergy, 56(5), pp.460-460. http://onlinelibrary.wiley.com/doi/10.1034/j.1398-9995.2001.056005460.x/full

Loblay, R.H. and Swain, A.R., 2006, 'Food Intolerance', Recent Advances in Clinical Nutrition, retrieved from www.nsw.gov.au.

O'Regan, G.M., Sandilands, A., McLean, W.I. and Irvine, A.D., 2009. Filaggrin in atopic dermatitis. Journal of Allergy and Clinical Immunology,124(3), pp.R2-R6.

Arreola, R., Quintero-Fabián, S., López-Roa, R.I., Flores-Gutiérrez, E.O., Reyes-Grajeda, J.P., Carrera-Quintanar, L. and Ortuño-Sahagún, D., 2015. Immunomodulation and anti-inflammatory effects of garlic compounds.Journal of immunology research, 2015.

https://nationaleczema.org/top-advances-in-eczema-research-in-2016/

https://www.allergy.org.au/patients/skin-allergy/eczema

https://www.ncbi.nlm.nih.gov/books/NBK279399/

https://www.medicalnewstoday.com/articles/318946.php